COMPLETE GUIDE TO GASTROINTESTINAL BLEEDING

A Comprehensive Handbook For Diagnosis, Treatment, Prevention Strategies, Essential Insights For Physicians, Surgeons, And Healthcare Professionals

DEHART HAIRSTON

© [DEHART HAIRSTON], [2024]

All rights reserved. No part of this publication may be reproduced, distributed, or transmitted in any form or by any means, including photocopying, recording, or other electronic or mechanical methods, without the prior written permission of the publisher, except in the case of brief quotations embodied in critical reviews and certain other noncommercial uses permitted by copyright law.

DISCLAIMER

This book's content is only intended for general informative purposes. At the time of writing, the author has taken every precaution to guarantee that the material is correct and current. Nevertheless, the author disclaims all explicit and implicit representations and guarantees about the availability, appropriateness, correctness, completeness, and usefulness of the material on these pages.

Since the author is not a licensed medical practitioner, the material in this book shouldn't be interpreted as medical advice. Before making any modifications to their diet, exercise regimen, or medical treatment, readers are urged to speak with a licensed healthcare provider.

Moreover, the author has no connection to any of the businesses, organizations, or people that are discussed in this book. Any mentions of goods, services, businesses, or people are purely informative and do not indicate endorsement or suggestion.

This book's content is entirely dependent on the author's expertise, study, and comprehension of the topic. Despite having taken reasonable care to offer correct information, the author disclaims all liability for any mistakes or omissions in the material as well as for any losses, harm, or damages resulting from using the information.

It is recommended that readers use their own judgment and discretion when applying the knowledge in this book to their own situations. The use or implementation of any material in this book may result in unfavorable repercussions, directly or indirectly, for which the author assumes no liability.

By reading this book, you agree to release and hold the author harmless from any claims, losses, liabilities, costs, or expenditures resulting from or related to the use of the information you get from it.

Table of Contents

CHAPTER 1 13
- Understanding Gastrointestinal Bleeding 13
- What Is Gastrointestinal Bleeding? 13
- Causes And Risk Factors 14
- Types Of Gastrointestinal Bleeding 15
- Signs And Symptoms 16

CHAPTER 2 19
- Anatomy And Physiology Of The Gastrointestinal Tract 19
- Overview Of The Gi Tract 19
- Functions Of Different Parts Of The Gi Tract 20
- Understanding Blood Supply To The Gi Tract 22

CHAPTER 3 25
- Diagnostic Approaches 25
- History Taking And Physical Examination 25
- Laboratory Tests 26
- Imaging Studies (Endoscopy, Colonoscopy, Angiography) 27
- Role Of Biopsy In Diagnosis 28

CHAPTER 4 31
- Initial Management 31

Stabilization Of The Patient 31
Fluid Resuscitation 32
Blood Transfusion 33
Pharmacological Interventions (Proton Pump Inhibitors, Octreotide) 34

CHAPTER 5 37
Endoscopic Interventions 37
Principles Of Endoscopy 37
Endoscopic Hemostasis Techniques (Clips, Bands, Thermal Methods) 38
Role Of Endoscopic Therapy In Different Types Of Bleeding 40

CHAPTER 6 43
Surgical Management 43
Indications For Surgery In Gastrointestinal Bleeding 43
Surgical Options (Resection, Ligation, Embolization) 45
Postoperative Care And Complications 46

CHAPTER 7 49
Pharmacological Therapy 49
Pharmacological Agents For Acute And Chronic Management 49

Acute Care 49

Chronic Care 50

Anticoagulants And Antiplatelet Agents
Management In Gi Bleeding 51

CHAPTER 8 55

Complications And Prognosis 55

Complications Of Gastrointestinal Bleeding
(Anemia, Rebleeding, Perforation).........................55

Anemia 55

Rebleeding..56

Breach 56

Factors Influencing Prognosis..................................57

Root Cause 57

Level of Blood Loss 58

Combined conditions 58

Age and General Health 59

Reaction to the Intervention...............................59

CHAPTER 9 61

Preventive Measures 61

Lifestyle Modifications..61

Screening Strategies For High-Risk Populations ...63

Role Of Prophylactic Medications 65

CHAPTER 10 67
Patient Education And Support 67
Importance Of Patient Education In Preventing
Recurrent Bleeding 67
Resources And Support Groups For Patients And
Caregivers 70
Follow-Up Care And Monitoring 72
CONCLUSION 75
THE END 78

ABOUT THIS BOOK

For anyone worried about their gastrointestinal health and medical experts, this book, "Gastrointestinal Bleeding," is an invaluable resource. Its thorough coverage covers all facets of gastrointestinal bleeding, including diagnosis techniques, treatment plans, and preventative measures, in addition to comprehending the origins and symptoms of the condition. Allow me to explain why this book is a must-have for your medical collection.

First of all, it provides a thorough examination of the basics of gastrointestinal bleeding in Chapter 1, guaranteeing a firm grasp of the illness. In Chapter 2, the architecture and physiology of the gastrointestinal tract are outlined. This helps readers understand how bleeding happens within this intricate system, which may help with diagnostic and treatment choices.

Chapter 3's diagnostic methodologies provide a comprehensive guide for medical professionals, including everything from physical examinations and history collection to sophisticated imaging scans and biopsy methods. In Chapter 4, the topic of first care is discussed. The need for timely stabilization, fluid resuscitation, and pharmaceutical therapies to save lives is emphasized.

The endoscopic procedures covered in Chapter 5 provide up-to-date hemostasis approaches that are customized to address various forms of bleeding. When endoscopic procedures are found to be inadequate, surgical management—which guides surgeons on indications, alternatives, and postoperative care—becomes crucial, as delineated in Chapter 6.

In-depth discussions of pharmacological treatment, complications, and prognosis may be found in Chapters 7 and 8, which provide a comprehensive grasp of acute and chronic care strategies. Crucially, Chapter 9 concentrates on preventive approaches, arming medical professionals and patients with information on lifestyle adjustments, screening techniques, and preventative drugs to lessen the chance of recurrent bleeding.

Finally, Chapter 10 highlights the need for patient support and education, acknowledging the critical role that patients and caregivers play in successfully treating gastrointestinal bleeding. This book guarantees comprehensive patient care outside of the professional context by providing resources, support groups, and advice on follow-up care.

In summary, "Gastrointestinal Bleeding" is more than just a book; it's an extensive manual that gives medical practitioners the information and resources they need to successfully handle every facet of gastrointestinal bleeding.

This book is an essential tool that you just cannot afford to ignore, regardless of your level of experience as a gastroenterologist or your status as a medical student looking to further your knowledge.

CHAPTER 1

Understanding Gastrointestinal Bleeding

What Is Gastrointestinal Bleeding?

Any kind of bleeding that happens inside the digestive system, which stretches from the mouth to the anus, is referred to as gastrointestinal bleeding, or GI bleeding for short. It may appear in several ways, ranging from little bleeding that can be missed to serious bleeding that has to be treated right once. Any portion of the digestive system, including the esophagus, stomach, small intestine, large intestine (colon), or rectum, might be the source of GI bleeding. For an early diagnosis and suitable treatment, it is essential to comprehend the forms, indications, and symptoms, as well as the underlying causes and risk factors, of gastrointestinal bleeding.

Causes And Risk Factors

Gastrointestinal bleeding may be caused by several things, from minor ailments to more severe illnesses. One of the main causes of GI bleeding is peptic ulcers, which are sores that form on the lining of the stomach or upper portion of the small intestine. Diverticulosis (the existence of tiny pouches in the colon), esophageal varices (enlarged veins in the esophagus), hemorrhoids (swollen veins in the rectum or anus), and gastritis (inflammation of the stomach lining) are other frequent reasons.

Some risk factors might make someone more likely to bleed internally. Advanced age, a history of gastrointestinal issues or surgeries, heavy alcohol use, frequent use of nonsteroidal anti-inflammatory drugs (NSAIDs) like ibuprofen or aspirin, smoking, and underlying medical conditions like blood clotting disorders or liver disease are some of these risk factors.

Types Of Gastrointestinal Bleeding

Depending on where the bleeding occurs in the digestive system, there are two primary categories of gastrointestinal bleeding: upper gastrointestinal bleeding (UGIB) and lower gastrointestinal bleeding (LGIB).

- **Lower Gastrointestinal Bleeding (UGIB):** This kind of bleeding usually affects the stomach, duodenum, or esophagus and takes place in the upper section of the digestive system (the first part of the small intestine). Gastritis, esophageal varices, peptic ulcers, and Mallory-Weiss tears—tears in the esophageal lining—are often cited as causes of upper gastrointestinal bleeding.

- **Lower Gastrointestinal Bleeding (LGIB):** This is the term for bleeding that comes from the colon, rectum, or anus, which are all located in the lower portion of the digestive system. Diverticulosis, hemorrhoids, colorectal polyps, inflammatory bowel illness (such as Crohn's disease or ulcerative colitis), and colorectal cancer are among the common causes of LGIB.

Signs And Symptoms

Depending on the extent and location of the bleeding, there may be a range of signs and symptoms associated with gastrointestinal bleeding. While some people may just have minor symptoms that go away on their own, others can need immediate medical attention. When there is GI bleeding, common signs and symptoms include:

- **Rectal Bleeding:** One of the most obvious signs of gastrointestinal bleeding is this.

Depending on where and how fast the bleeding is occurring, the blood in the stool may look bright red, maroon, or black. Black, tarry feces are called melena, and they often signify upper gastrointestinal hemorrhage.

- **Vomiting Blood:** Also referred to as hematemesis, vomiting blood may happen as a result of bleeding in the upper small intestine, stomach, or esophagus. If the blood has been partly digested, it may look coffee-ground or brilliant crimson when it is vomited.

- **Stomach Pain or Discomfort:** Depending on the underlying reason for the bleeding, some people may have stomach pain or discomfort, which may vary in degree. GI bleeding may cause localized or widespread abdominal discomfort, which might become worse when you eat or move in certain ways.

- **Weakness and Fatigue:** Anemia, which is defined as a low red blood cell count, may result from severe or chronic gastrointestinal bleeding. Symptoms of anemia include weakness, exhaustion, breathing difficulties, and pale complexion.

- **Dizziness or fainting:** Severe GI bleeding may cause significant blood loss, which can lower blood pressure and oxygen supply to the brain. This can cause symptoms like lightheadedness, dizziness, or fainting (syncope).

- **Modifications to Bowel Habits:** Gastrointestinal bleeding may result in constipation or diarrhea. Sometimes people feel like they need to go to the bathroom right away.

If you see any signs or symptoms of gastrointestinal bleeding, you should consult a doctor right away since timely diagnosis and treatment may help avoid problems and improve results.

CHAPTER 2

Anatomy And Physiology Of The Gastrointestinal Tract

Overview Of The Gi Tract

The digestive tract, often known as the gastrointestinal (GI) tract, is a multifaceted system that helps the body break down food, absorb nutrients, and get rid of waste. It encompasses many organs and starts at the mouth and finishes at the anus. It is essential to comprehend the GI tract's architecture and physiology to properly diagnose and treat gastrointestinal bleeding.

The mouth, esophagus, stomach, small intestine, large intestine (colon), rectum, and anus are the six primary sections that make up the GI tract. Each component has a distinct function throughout the digestive process.

For instance, food enters the mouth by chewing, where it starts the process of mechanical and chemical digestion through salivation. Using peristaltic contractions, the esophagus is a muscular tube that carries food from the mouth to the stomach.

Functions Of Different Parts Of The Gi Tract

1. Mouth: Mastication (chewing) and the preliminary breakdown of food are done in the mouth, which serves as the entrance point of the digestive system. Enzymes found in saliva, which is secreted by salivary glands, initiate the breakdown of carbohydrates.

2. Stomach: The stomach completes the digestion process that was started in the mouth and acts as a temporary storage space for meals. Food particles are further broken down by gastric fluids, which include enzymes and hydrochloric acid, forming chyme, a semi-liquid material.

3. Small Intestine: The bulk of nutritional absorption takes place in the small intestine. It is separated into the ileum, jejunum, and duodenum. Villi and microvilli lining the walls of the small intestine enhance the surface area that is accessible for absorption.

4. Large Intestine: The colon, also known as the large intestine, forms solid waste (feces) for excretion after absorbing water and electrolytes from undigested food. Additionally, it is home to a large colony of helpful bacteria that assist in vitamin production and digestion.

5. Rectum and Anus: During defecation, the rectum holds on to waste materials until they are released from the body via the anus.

It is crucial to comprehend how each component of the GI tract works to identify anomalies that might result in gastrointestinal bleeding.

Understanding Blood Supply To The Gi Tract

The superior, inferior, and celiac mesenteric arteries are among the branches of the abdominal aorta that give blood to the gastrointestinal system. These arteries divide to deliver blood to various parts of the gastrointestinal system, guaranteeing that every organ gets enough nutrition and oxygen.

1. Celiac Artery: The pancreas, stomach, liver, and spleen get blood supply from the celiac artery, which divides from the abdominal aorta.

2. The ileum, duodenum, and jejunum in the small intestine and the proximal two-thirds of the transverse colon in the large intestine get blood supply from the Superior Mesenteric Artery (SMA),

which emerges from the abdominal aorta slightly below the celiac artery.

3. The third main branch of the abdominal aorta, the inferior mesenteric artery (IMA), provides blood to the distal third of the sigmoid colon, transverse colon, descending colon, and rectum.

It is essential to comprehend the blood supply to the gastrointestinal tract since disturbances in blood flow may induce ischemia, or absence of blood flow, which may cause tissue injury or gastrointestinal bleeding. Serious consequences may arise from disorders that impair blood flow to the gastrointestinal system, such as embolism, thrombosis, or atherosclerosis.

In summary, accurate diagnosis and treatment of gastrointestinal bleeding depend on a thorough knowledge of the architecture, physiology, and blood supply of the GI tract.

Healthcare workers may improve patient care and outcomes by properly evaluating and treating patients with GI bleeding by knowing the blood supply and functioning of the various regions of the GI tract.

CHAPTER 3

Diagnostic Approaches

History Taking And Physical Examination

One of the most important steps in identifying gastrointestinal bleeding is collecting a complete history and doing a physical examination. Important hints about potential bleeding causes may be found in the patient's medical history. To assist narrow down the possible underlying illnesses, one might ask about recent trauma, medication usage, alcohol intake, and history of gastrointestinal issues.

Healthcare professionals may search for indications of bleeding during the physical examination, such as pallor, low blood pressure, an elevated heart rate, or discomfort in the abdomen. Upon rectal examination, anomalies such as blood in the stool may be discovered.

These results, in conjunction with the patient's medical history and symptoms, might direct further diagnostic studies.

Laboratory Tests

An important part of evaluating gastrointestinal bleeding is laboratory testing. Anemia is often detected by blood tests like the complete blood count (CBC), especially in individuals who have had severe blood loss. Tests to measure coagulation parameters may also be carried out to check for coagulopathies brought on by medications or bleeding problems.

Furthermore, even in cases when minute quantities of blood in the feces are invisible to the unaided eye, stool tests like the fecal occult blood test (FOBT) and fecal immunochemical test (FIT) may identify them.

These non-invasive examinations are often used as preliminary screening methods to identify gastrointestinal hemorrhage.

Imaging Studies (Endoscopy, Colonoscopy, Angiography)

Finding the cause and degree of gastrointestinal bleeding requires the use of imaging tests. Commonly used techniques that provide direct sight of the gastrointestinal system include endoscopy and colonoscopy. While a colonoscopy assesses the colon and terminal ileum, an upper endoscopy (also known as an esophagogastroduodenoscopy or EGD) looks at the esophagus, stomach, and duodenum.

The medical professional might find bleeding causes including polyps, tumors, ulcers, and arteriovenous malformations during these operations. Furthermore, endoscopic procedures like cauterization or clipping may be used to halt ongoing bleeding or stop such events in the future.

Angiography may be used if an endoscopy or colonoscopy is unable to identify the source of the bleeding. To see any aberrant blood flow, an angiography involves injecting contrast dye into the blood arteries. It is especially helpful in identifying bleeding from arterial causes, such as tumor-induced arterial bleeding or gastrointestinal arteriovenous malformations.

Role Of Biopsy In Diagnosis

When endoscopic results are unclear or a precise diagnosis is required for the right course of treatment, a biopsy is an essential diagnostic tool for gastrointestinal bleeding. Tissue samples (biopsies) may be taken from suspected lesions or regions of mucosal abnormalities during an endoscopy or colonoscopy.

A pathologist then looks at these biopsy samples under a microscope to look for any underlying pathology, such as infection, inflammation, dysplasia, or cancer. The biopsy's findings may provide important information that helps identify the source of the bleeding and direct further care, such as starting certain medications or monitoring procedures.

To successfully evaluate gastrointestinal bleeding, a thorough diagnostic strategy that includes laboratory testing, imaging investigations, physical examination, history collection, and biopsy is necessary. Combining these technologies allows medical professionals to precisely pinpoint the bleeding cause and apply the right treatments to properly manage the patient's condition.

CHAPTER 4

Initial Management

Stabilization Of The Patient

The first thing to do when a patient has gastrointestinal bleeding (GIB) is to stabilize them. This entails evaluating the patient's vital signs, including oxygen saturation, heart rate, blood pressure, and breathing rate. To detect symptoms of shock or severe blood loss, such as pallor, diaphoresis, or changed mental state, a complete physical examination is essential.

Securing the patient's airway and maintaining proper breathing and oxygenation are frequently the first steps toward stabilization. Fluid resuscitation requires immediate intravenous access if the patient is hypotensive or in shock. Large-bore peripheral intravenous lines or even central venous access may be required in extreme situations when there is suspicion of continuous bleeding.

Furthermore, ideal patient positioning—typically supine with legs raised—can enhance cardiac output and venous return. Throughout stabilization, it is critical to keep an eye out for any indications of continued bleeding, such as melena (black, tarry stools) or hematemesis (blood in the vomit).

Fluid Resuscitation

The foundation of the first line of treatment for gastrointestinal bleeding is fluid resuscitation. Restoring intravascular volume and enhancing tissue perfusion will lessen the chance of shock and organ failure. Usually, the first treatments are isotonic crystalloid solutions, such as plain saline or lactated Ringer's solution.

The degree of bleeding and the patient's hemodynamic state determine how much fluid is needed. Fluid replacement treatment is guided by continuous monitoring of vital signs, urine output, and laboratory markers such as hematocrit and hemoglobin levels. Aggressive fluid resuscitation may be required in situations of severe bleeding to keep important organs perfused until final therapy can be started.

Blood Transfusion

Blood transfusions could be required in situations of severe gastrointestinal bleeding or persistent hemorrhage to replenish lost red blood cells and regain the body's ability to transport oxygen. Transfusion thresholds vary according to the patient's age, comorbidities, and hemodynamic stability, among other variables.

To keep hemoglobin levels over a certain threshold—often 7-8 g/dL in stable patients and higher in those with active bleeding or hemodynamic instability—packed red blood cells, or PRBCs, are typically transfused. Transfusions of fresh frozen plasma and platelets may also be necessary in patients with thrombocytopenia or coagulopathy brought on by acute blood loss.

Pharmacological Interventions (Proton Pump Inhibitors, Octreotide)

The early treatment of gastrointestinal bleeding heavily relies on pharmacological therapies. Omeprazole and pantoprazole are two examples of proton pump inhibitors (PPIs), which are often used to lower stomach acid output and encourage mucosal repair. When there is upper gastrointestinal bleeding, they are especially helpful since acid suppression may stop the bleeding from returning and assist in stabilizing the clot.

Another pharmaceutical treatment for gastrointestinal bleeding is octreotide, an analog of somatostatin that is particularly useful when variceal hemorrhage is present. It lowers portal hypertension and the risk of variceal rupture by lowering splanchnic blood flow and preventing the production of vasoactive chemicals.

These pharmacological therapies are usually given intravenously, and based on the patient's reaction to therapy and the underlying cause of the bleeding, they may be maintained as part of the continuing care plan. Throughout the first phase of therapy, careful observation for side effects and frequent reevaluations of the patient's clinical state is necessary.

CHAPTER 5

Endoscopic Interventions

Principles Of Endoscopy

An essential tool for identifying and managing gastrointestinal bleeding (GIB) is endoscopy. To see the gastrointestinal system, a flexible tube equipped with a camera and light source must be inserted via the mouth or rectum. Accurately locating the bleeding source is the main objective.

The endoscopist gently moves the scope through the esophagus, stomach, and small intestine (for upper GIB) or the colon and rectum (for lower GIB) during an endoscopic operation. The camera's photos provide real-time imaging of the mucosa of the gastrointestinal tract, making it possible to identify anomalies such as ulcers, varices, or lesions that could be causing bleeding.

To fully inspect the gastrointestinal system, the endoscope must be controlled and maneuvered precisely. The endoscopist has to be skilled at using the scope to maneuver around curves and bends while causing the patient as little pain as possible.

Additionally, the endoscopic suite has several tools and accessories that help with procedures like hemostasis. These might consist of cautery devices, bands, clips, and probes, each with a distinct function in the treatment of bleeding lesions.

Endoscopic Hemostasis Techniques (Clips, Bands, Thermal Methods)

Endoscopic hemostasis describes the actions taken during an endoscopy to halt bleeding from gastrointestinal tract lesions. The decision between various procedures is contingent upon several criteria, including the precise location and kind of bleeding lesion, the patient's clinical status, and the endoscopist's level of skill.

1. Endoscopic clips are tiny metallic devices that are used to mechanically seal ulcers or bleeding arteries. Through a specific clip applicator that is fastened to the endoscope, they are discharged. The clip efficiently seals the lesion and stops the bleeding once it is placed over the bleeding location and released.

2. **Bands:** Hemorrhoids or esophageal varices, which are prone to bleeding, are often treated by band ligation. The base of the varix or hemorrhoidal tissue is wrapped with a rubber band to induce ischemia and necrosis, which stops the bleeding.

3. **Thermal Techniques:** These include a range of modalities, including heater probes, argon plasma coagulation (APC), and electrocautery. These techniques cauterize tissue or bleeding vessels

using heat radiation to stop the bleeding completely.

Every hemostatic method has benefits and drawbacks, therefore the endoscopist must evaluate the particular clinical situation to choose the best course of action.

Role Of Endoscopic Therapy In Different Types Of Bleeding

In the treatment of many gastrointestinal bleeding disorders, such as upper and lower GIB, as well as particular diseases including peptic ulcers, variceal hemorrhage, and angiodysplasia, endoscopic therapy is essential.

1. Upper GIB: Bleeding ulcers, erosions, and varices in the upper gastrointestinal tract are often treated with endoscopic treatment. To achieve hemostasis and stop rebleeding, endoscopic hemostasis procedures including banding, clipping, and thermal coagulation work well.

2. Lower GIB: Diverticula, angiodysplasia, and colonic ulcers are among the lesions that endoscopy may assist diagnose and treating when there is lower gastrointestinal bleeding. By immediately applying hemostatic therapies to the bleeding source, less invasive procedures are required.

3. Variceal Bleeding: The main therapy for esophageal varices, which often result in upper GIB in individuals with liver cirrhosis, is endoscopic band ligation. Endoscopic treatment improves patient outcomes by reducing the risk of variceal rebleeding by ligating the varices.

4. Angiodysplasia: Recurrent bleeding is a common occurrence in gastrointestinal tract angiodysplastic lesions. These aberrant blood vessels may be destroyed by endoscopic methods like thermal coagulation or injectable sclerotherapy to stop further bleeding episodes.

All things considered, endoscopic treatment provides a less intrusive and successful method of controlling gastrointestinal bleeding, with the ability to achieve hemostasis, avert complications, and enhance patient survival.

CHAPTER 6

Surgical Management

Indications For Surgery In Gastrointestinal Bleeding

When it comes to gastrointestinal bleeding, surgery is considered when all other measures have failed to stop the bleeding or when the bleeding cause is thought to be surgically accessible. Several signs indicate whether surgery is necessary:

Persistent Bleeding: Surgery may be required to directly address the bleeding cause if bleeding persists after conservative measures such as medication or endoscopic procedures. This is often the case when there is a significant or persistent bleeding that is unresponsive to other forms of treatment.

Hemodynamic instability: Surgery may be necessary to halt the bleeding and stabilize the patient's health when a patient has considerable blood loss that results in unstable vital signs like low blood pressure or a fast heartbeat.

Failure of Endoscopic Intervention: Surgery can be necessary if endoscopic treatments are unable to stop the bleeding. Usually, the first line of treatment is endoscopy, but surgery may be required if it doesn't work or if the bleeding is too severe.

Suspected or Verified Structural Abnormalities: Vascular malformations, cancers, and ulcers are examples of structural abnormalities that may cause gastrointestinal bleeding. To fix or eliminate these anomalies and stop the bleeding, surgery becomes essential.

Recurrent Bleeding: Surgery may be suggested to treat the underlying cause and stop further episodes if a patient has severe or frequent gastrointestinal bleeding episodes that occur repeatedly.

Specific diseases: Depending on the kind of bleeding and the anatomy involved, certain diseases, such as major lower gastrointestinal bleeding or bleeding from Meckel's diverticulum, may need surgical intervention.

Surgical Options (Resection, Ligation, Embolization)

Resection is the process of removing the damaged area of the digestive system, such as a section of the intestine that has an ulcer or bleeding tumor in it. The goal of this treatment is to stop the bleeding and get the digestive system back to normal.

Ligation: By cutting off or closing the blood arteries feeding the injured region, this method stops bleeding. During surgery, this technique is often used to stop bleeding from tiny blood arteries or arteriovenous malformations.

Embolization: An injectable coil or particle is injected into the blood arteries feeding the bleeding spot by a radiologist during this minimally invasive technique to stop the blood flow. This method works very well for stopping bleeding from tumors or vascular abnormalities.

Postoperative Care And Complications

For the best recovery and to avoid complications, extensive postoperative care is essential after surgical therapy for gastrointestinal bleeding. This comprises:

Monitoring: In the early postoperative phase, careful observation of hemoglobin levels, vital signs, and indications of bleeding or infection is crucial. Ongoing evaluation facilitates early problem detection and timely response.

Pain treatment: To guarantee patient comfort and speed up recovery, adequate pain management is crucial. The method used to provide pain medicine may vary depending on the kind of operation done, including oral, intravenous, and other methods.

Nutritional Support: A patient's capacity to eat and absorb nutrients correctly may be impacted by gastrointestinal surgery. During the healing process, nutritional support—such as feeding tubes or intravenous fluids—might be required to maintain sufficient nourishment.

Preventive measures should be taken to avoid problems including infection, deep vein thrombosis, or pulmonary embolism. Prophylactic antibiotics, early mobilization, and compression stockings to enhance circulation are a few examples of this.

Follow-Up Care: To track their development, identify any issues, and modify their treatment plan as necessary, patients should have routine follow-up care. This might include follow-up imaging examinations, endoscopic assessments, or expert consultations.

After gastrointestinal surgery, anesthesia-related problems, bowel blockage, bleeding, infection, and anastomotic leaks are possible after-effects. Timely identification and treatment of these issues are crucial in guaranteeing positive results and encouraging patient recuperation.

When conservative methods are ineffective in controlling bleeding or when there are particular reasons for surgical intervention, surgical therapy of gastrointestinal bleeding is recommended.

CHAPTER 7

Pharmacological Therapy

Pharmacological Agents For Acute And Chronic Management

Pharmacological treatment is essential for the management of gastrointestinal (GI) bleeding since it provides alternatives for both acute and long-term care. These pharmaceuticals are intended to treat bleeding in several ways, such as coagulation, inflammation, and ulcer healing.

Acute Care

The main objective of treating acute gastrointestinal bleeding is to stabilize the patient's state while quickly stopping the bleeding. In this case, the goal of pharmacotherapy is to establish hemostasis and stop further bleeding. Proton pump inhibitors are a major family of medications used in acute care

(PPIs). PPIs function by decreasing the production of stomach acid, which may aid in stabilizing bleeding ulcers and accelerating their recovery.

Vasoconstrictors, such as terlipressin and octreotide, are another crucial element of acute treatment. These medications function by narrowing blood arteries, which reduces blood flow to the area of bleeding and aids in hemostasis. Furthermore, the release of several hormones and peptides involved in the control of blood flow and stomach acid secretion may be suppressed by somatostatin analogs such as octreotide.

Chronic Care

A different strategy is needed for chronic GI bleeding than for acute episodes. When it comes to chronic care, the emphasis switches to controlling underlying diseases that cause bleeding and avoiding recurring bleeding episodes. In this context, pharmacotherapy often refers to the long-term use of drugs meant to lower bleeding risk and encourage mucosal repair.

H2-receptor antagonists are a major family of medications used in chronic treatment. By preventing histamine from acting on stomach H2 receptors, these medications lessen the production of gastric acid and speed up the healing of ulcers. Prostaglandin analogs, such as misoprostol, may also be helpful by strengthening mucosal defense and encouraging the development of a barrier to protect the stomach.

Anticoagulants And Antiplatelet Agents Management In Gi Bleeding

The risks and advantages of maintaining or stopping anticoagulants and antiplatelet medicines must be carefully considered when managing gastrointestinal bleeding in individuals on these drugs. Patients with a variety of cardiovascular and thrombotic diseases are often prescribed anticoagulants, such as warfarin, dabigatran, rivaroxaban, and apixaban, to avoid thromboembolic events.

Reversal medications may be required in situations of acute gastrointestinal bleeding in individuals taking anticoagulants to quickly stop the anticoagulant's effects and stop bleeding. For example, vitamin K may be used to counteract the effects of warfarin, and particular antidotes such as andexanet alfa for factor Xa inhibitors or idarucizumab for dabigatran can be used for targeted reversal.

In the case of GI bleeding, patients using antiplatelet medications like ticagrelor, clopidogrel, prasugrel, or aspirin may also need specialized care techniques. Sometimes, particularly when the bleeding is serious or life-threatening, it may be essential to temporarily stop using these medications to lower the chance of the bleeding continuing.

Medication treatment is essential for managing gastrointestinal bleeding in both acute and long-term situations. Healthcare professionals may make well-informed choices to maximize patient outcomes while lowering the risk of consequences by having a thorough understanding of the many kinds of medications used, their mechanisms of action, and their indications.

CHAPTER 8

Complications And Prognosis

Complications Of Gastrointestinal Bleeding (Anemia, Rebleeding, Perforation)

Anemia

Because of the blood loss, anemia is one of the main effects of gastrointestinal bleeding. The body's iron reserves are depleted by blood loss from the gastrointestinal system, which lowers hemoglobin and red blood cell counts. Pale complexion, weakness, exhaustion, and dyspnea are some of the signs of anemia. If treatment is not received, it may potentially cause organ damage in extreme circumstances. To treat anemia, the bleeding cause must be closed, and low iron levels must be restored by transfusions or supplements.

Rebleeding

Another major worry in situations of gastrointestinal bleeding is rebleeding. There is a chance that the bleeding may return even after the first round of medication. This may occur for several reasons, such as the bleeding source not fully stopping, the development of new lesions, or the continued presence of underlying disorders that increase the risk of bleeding. Depending on the severity of the recurrence, rebleeding may need further treatments, including repeat endoscopic procedures or surgery, and may cause more difficulties.

Breach

There is a chance of perforation in some gastrointestinal bleeding instances, especially those involving ulcers or erosions. A perforation is a hole in the gastrointestinal wall that allows stomach contents to seep into the abdominal cavity. If left untreated, this may lead to severe abdominal discomfort, fever, peritonitis symptoms, and potentially fatal consequences including septic shock. To fix the hole and stop further consequences, perforation frequently needs surgical intervention as well as rapid medical treatment.

Factors Influencing Prognosis

Root Cause

The underlying source of the bleeding has a substantial impact on the prognosis of gastrointestinal hemorrhage. The prognosis for diseases including peptic ulcers, esophageal varices, colon cancer, and inflammatory bowel disease might vary depending on the illness's stage, response to therapy, and coexisting conditions. Early detection and treatment of the underlying cause may enhance the prognosis and lower the chance of complications.

Level of Blood Loss

One of the most important factors in deciding prognosis is the degree of gastrointestinal bleeding. If massive bleeding is not treated quickly, it may result in shock, organ failure, and hemodynamic instability. On the other hand, mild bleeding episodes may improve with cautious therapy or resolve on their own. Improving results and lowering death rates need a quick assessment of the extent of bleeding and prompt action.

Combined conditions

The prognosis of gastrointestinal bleeding may be greatly impacted by the existence of underlying medical problems. Individuals who suffer from concomitant conditions such as coagulopathies, liver cirrhosis, chronic renal disease, or cardiovascular disease may be more susceptible to complications and death. To maximize results and lower the chance of unfavorable events, it is important to manage these comorbidities in addition to gastrointestinal bleeding.

Age and General Health

Guterer bleeding prognosis is also affected by age and general health. Patients who are elderly or have substantial comorbidities may have lesser physiological reserves, making them more vulnerable to problems or delayed healing. On the other hand, those who are younger and in better condition could have a better prognosis and react better to therapy. To maximize results and improve prognosis, the therapeutic strategy must be customized based on the unique features of each patient.

Reaction to the Intervention

Lastly, an important consideration in assessing prognosis is the patient's reaction to therapy. In contrast to patients who suffer treatment failure or recurrent bleeding, those who react well to early therapies, such as endoscopic therapy, medicinal management, or surgical intervention, have a better prognosis. Reducing the likelihood of problems and improving outcomes need quick management strategy adjustments as well as close monitoring of patient's responses to therapy.

CHAPTER 9

Preventive Measures

Lifestyle Modifications

Making changes to one's lifestyle is essential to halting gastrointestinal bleeding. These modifications are intended to improve general digestive health and lower the risk factors related to this illness. Adopting a balanced diet high in fruits, vegetables, and fiber while reducing the consumption of processed foods, saturated fats, and spicy meals is one of the main lifestyle changes. This dietary strategy helps maintain a healthy weight, which is crucial since obesity raises the risk of gastrointestinal problems, in addition to promoting good digestion.

In addition, reducing alcohol intake and giving up smoking are crucial measures in avoiding gastrointestinal bleeding. The lining of the digestive system may become irritated by smoking and excessive alcohol use, which increases the risk of bleeding ulcers. People may drastically reduce their likelihood of experiencing gastrointestinal issues by giving up these practices.

Another essential element of changing one's lifestyle to stop gastrointestinal bleeding is regular exercise. Physical exercise supports immune system strength, good weight maintenance, and improved blood circulation. Exercise also helps lower stress levels, which is beneficial since stress has been connected to several digestive issues, such as gastritis and peptic ulcers.

To sum up, lifestyle changes including eating a balanced diet, giving up smoking, consuming alcohol in moderation, and exercising often are important ways to avoid gastrointestinal bleeding. The likelihood of acquiring this dangerous medical condition may be considerably decreased by making some easy but effective modifications.

Screening Strategies For High-Risk Populations

To identify gastrointestinal bleeding early and provide timely intervention and treatment, screening measures for high-risk patients are crucial. A history of gastrointestinal illnesses, such as peptic ulcers, gastrointestinal malignancies, or inflammatory bowel disease, as well as specific risk factors, such as advanced age or a family history of gastrointestinal problems, identify people as high-risk.

Endoscopy is one of the main screening techniques used on high-risk groups. To inspect the lining of the digestive system, a flexible tube with a camera attached is used in this technique. Endoscopy enables medical professionals to respond appropriately by detecting anomalies such as ulcers, polyps, or bleeding spots.

For certain high-risk patients, additional screening procedures such as fecal occult blood tests (FOBT) and fecal immunochemical testing (FIT) may be advised in addition to endoscopy. The presence of blood in the stool, which may be an indication of gastrointestinal bleeding, is detected by these non-invasive tests. These tests may not provide as much specific information about the bleeding cause as endoscopy, although they are less intrusive than that procedure.

Frequent screening is essential for early diagnosis and management in high-risk groups. Early detection of gastrointestinal bleeding allows medical professionals to start the right therapy early on, preventing complications and improving patient outcomes.

Role Of Prophylactic Medications

When it comes to those who are at a higher risk of bleeding from the gastrointestinal tract because of certain medical problems or drugs, preventative measures are quite important. By shielding the lining of the digestive system or lowering the formation of stomach acid, these drugs are intended to lower the risk of ulcers and bleeding.

Proton pump inhibitors are one kind of preventive medicine that is often used (PPIs). PPIs function by preventing the stomach from producing acid, which lowers the risk of ulcers and bleeding in the upper gastrointestinal tract and stomach. People who use nonsteroidal anti-inflammatory medicines (NSAIDs), which raise the risk of gastrointestinal problems, are often administered these treatments.

H2 receptor antagonists are another family of preventive drugs that lessen the formation of stomach acid and may help stop bleeding and ulcers. When using PPIs, these drugs are sometimes combined for the benefit of those who are more susceptible to gastrointestinal problems.

To shield the lining of the stomach and intestines from harm from acid and other irritants, doctors may also prescribe cytoprotective drugs like sucralfate in addition to acid-reducing ones. These drugs create a layer of defense over sores or ulcers, enabling them to heal and stopping further bleeding.

All things considered, preventive drugs are essential for avoiding gastrointestinal bleeding in high-risk patients. These drugs may help lower the risk of ulcers and bleeding by decreasing the production of stomach acid or shielding the lining of the digestive system, which will eventually improve patient outcomes.

CHAPTER 10

Patient Education And Support

Importance Of Patient Education In Preventing Recurrent Bleeding

To stop gastrointestinal bleeding from occurring again, patient education is essential. Patients get the ability to actively engage in their healthcare journey when they are informed about their disease, available treatments, and preventative actions. This empowerment eventually lowers the likelihood of repeated bleeding episodes by improving adherence to treatment strategies, modifying lifestyle choices, and identifying warning signals early.

Knowing the underlying causes of gastrointestinal bleeding is an important part of patient education. Whether they suffer from peptic ulcers, esophageal varices, inflammatory bowel disease, or other gastrointestinal problems, patients must understand the variables that lead to their condition. Patients may reduce the chance of recurrence by making educated decisions regarding their food, medicines, and way of life by being aware of these factors.

Additionally, it is critical to teach patients the value of adhering to their prescription regimen. Aspirin, anticoagulants, and nonsteroidal anti-inflammatory medications (NSAIDs) are linked to a high number of episodes of gastrointestinal bleeding. Patients must be aware of the possible side effects of these drugs and how crucial it is to take them exactly as directed. Healthcare professionals should also talk to patients about adjunct therapy or other drugs that have a reduced risk of bleeding.

Making changes to one's lifestyle is also essential for avoiding repeated bleeding. Patients must be informed about the effects of smoking, drinking alcohol, and following certain dietary guidelines on their digestive systems. The risk of recurrence may be greatly decreased by promoting a balanced diet high in fruits, vegetables, and fiber and minimizing processed foods and alcohol.

Furthermore, warning signals of recurrent bleeding should be identified as part of patient education. Abdominal discomfort, dizziness, blood in the vomit, black, tarry stools, and other symptoms should all be treated medically right away. Enabling patients to identify these symptoms early on allows medical professionals to take quick action, perhaps averting problems and hospital stays.

In conclusion, patient education aims to enable individuals to take charge of their health rather than only dispensing information. Patients may lower the risk of recurring bleeding episodes and improve their quality of life by learning the causes of gastrointestinal bleeding, following treatment programs, changing their lifestyle, and identifying warning signals.

Resources And Support Groups For Patients And Caregivers

For both patients and caretakers, managing gastrointestinal bleeding may be very challenging. Thankfully, there are many tools and support systems accessible to provide direction, knowledge, and psychological support all along the way.

Patient advocacy groups that focus on gastrointestinal health are a useful resource. These groups often include instructional resources, discussion boards on the internet, and hotlines manned by individuals with expertise who may respond to inquiries and give advice. The National Digestive Diseases Information Clearinghouse (NDDIC), the Crohn's & Colitis Foundation, and the

American Gastroenterological Association (AGA) are a few examples.

Furthermore, a lot of medical centers and hospitals have support groups designed especially for patients with gastrointestinal bleeding and the people who care for them. These support groups provide people with a safe place to talk about their challenges, ask questions, and get advice from those who have been there before. Making connections with others who are going through similar things may be very reassuring and powerful.

In addition, healthcare professionals are essential in helping patients and caregivers find the right resources and support services. Referrals to dietitians, social workers, psychologists, and other experts who can handle particular requirements and difficulties associated with gastrointestinal bleeding may be made by them.

In general, patients and caregivers navigating the complications of gastrointestinal bleeding may benefit from the emotional support, important knowledge, and reduced feelings of isolation that come from accessing resources and support groups.

Follow-Up Care And Monitoring

To manage gastrointestinal bleeding and lower the chance of recurrence, monitoring, and follow-up treatment are crucial. Patients should schedule routine follow-up appointments with their healthcare provider following an initial bleeding episode to evaluate their condition, track the effectiveness of treatment, and look for any indications of complications or recurrence.

Healthcare professionals often conduct physical examinations, go over lab results, and suggest imaging tests or endoscopic procedures to assess the gastrointestinal tract during follow-up visits.

These evaluations assist in locating any underlying issues or problems that might call for medical attention.

Managing medications is another essential component of post-treatment care. Depending on the patient's response and any changes in their condition, medical professionals may change the medications they prescribe, change the dosages, or prescribe additional therapies. Patients must notify their healthcare provider as soon as they experience any new symptoms or side effects.

Follow-up care often involves lifestyle counseling and support in addition to medical management. To enhance digestive health and lower the risk of recurrent bleeding, healthcare professionals can provide advice on diet changes, exercise routines, quitting smoking, and alcohol reduction tactics.

Moreover, long-term monitoring may be necessary for patients with a history of gastrointestinal bleeding to identify early indicators of recurrence. This may entail surveillance endoscopies to examine the gastrointestinal mucosa for indications of inflammation, ulcers, or other anomalies, as well as routine blood tests to check for anemia or occult blood in the stool.

All things considered, effective management of gastrointestinal bleeding, improving treatment outcomes, and lowering the risk of complications and recurrent bleeding episodes depend on routine follow-up care and monitoring. Patients can protect their digestive health and enhance their general well-being by being proactive in their follow-up appointments and maintaining active communication with their healthcare providers.

CONCLUSION

To sum up, gastrointestinal bleeding is a serious medical issue that needs to be diagnosed as soon as possible and treated appropriately to reduce the risk of complications and enhance patient outcomes. We have covered a variety of gastrointestinal bleeding causes, symptoms, diagnosis techniques, and treatment options during this talk.

First and foremost, it's important to understand that many different conditions can cause bleeding in the gastrointestinal tract, from benign conditions like hemorrhoids to more serious problems like peptic ulcers, gastrointestinal cancers, or vascular abnormalities. This emphasizes how crucial it is to obtain a thorough medical history, perform a physical examination, and order diagnostic tests such as endoscopy, imaging studies, and laboratory investigations to precisely identify the source and location of bleeding.

Following a diagnosis, the course of treatment for gastrointestinal bleeding is determined by several variables, such as the extent of the bleeding, the underlying cause, and the general health of the patient. Acute interventions can include pharmacological therapies like proton pump inhibitors or vasoconstrictors to control bleeding and stabilize the patient, in addition to resuscitative measures like blood transfusions and fluid replacement. Hemostatic techniques, injection therapy, thermal coagulation, and hemostatic clipping can be used when endoscopic intervention is a viable option.

Long-term management approaches for recurrent or chronic bleeding may involve lifestyle changes, medication to relieve symptoms, and, in certain situations, minimally invasive or surgical procedures to address the underlying pathology. Close observation and follow-up care are also necessary to evaluate the effectiveness of treatment, identify complications, and modify management strategies as necessary.

In conclusion, the comprehensive management of gastrointestinal bleeding necessitates a multidisciplinary approach involving surgeons, hematologists, gastroenterologists, and other medical specialists. Clinicians can improve the quality of life and optimize patient outcomes by utilizing a customized treatment plan, prompt interventions, and precise diagnosis.

THE END

www.ingramcontent.com/pod-product-compliance
Lightning Source LLC
Chambersburg PA
CBHW070317230526
45470CB00002B/918